Intermittent Fasting

Burn Fat, Lose Weight,

and Become Energetic and

Happy

The following eBook is reproduced below with the goal of providing information that is as accurate and reliable as possible. Regardless, purchasing this eBook can be seen as consent to the fact that both the publisher and the author of this book are in no way experts on the topics discussed within and that any recommendations or suggestions that are made herein are for entertainment purposes only. Professionals should be consulted as needed prior to undertaking any of the action endorsed herein.

This declaration is deemed fair and valid by both the American Bar Association and the Committee of Publishers Association and is legally binding throughout the United States.

Furthermore, the transmission, duplication, or reproduction of any of the following work including specific information will be considered an illegal act irrespective of if it is done electronically or in print. This extends to creating a secondary or tertiary copy of the work or a recorded copy

Table of Contents

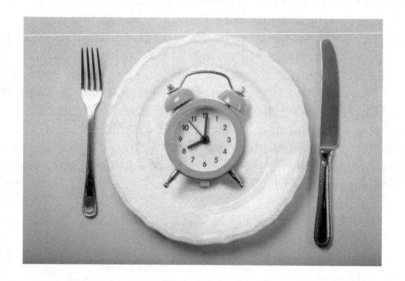

Introduction

Congratulations on purchasing this book, and thank you for doing so. The world of dieting is growing increasingly chaotic. Downloading this book is the first step that you can take towards doing something about healthy dieting. The first step will not always be the easiest, which is why the information you will find in the following chapters is so important to take to heart, as they are not concepts that can be put into action immediately. If you file these concepts away for when you need them, when the time comes to actually use them, you will be glad you have them at hand.

The following chapters will discuss the primary preparedness principles that you will need to consider if you ever hope to really lose weight and gain health through intermittent fasting. This means that you will want to consider the quality of your food, including the potential issues raised by their quality, how they can best be utilized in a meal, as well as various tools you might need to keep your mind focused on the task at hand.

With quality out of the way, you will then learn everything you need to know about preparing a wide variety of foods, including common fruit and vegetable, along with less common dishes as well. Rounding out the three primary requirements for successful dieting, you will then learn about crucial food storage principles and what they will mean for you. Finally, you will learn how building a diet plan is likely the best choice for realizing all your hard work.

We are happy to welcome you to the world of the intermittent fasting diet and to help you lose weight, change your life, and become a healthier person.

Chapter 1: Fasting: An Interesting Idea

The recipe for living long and healthy could be reducing the protein intake: but what happens to our body with semi-fast regimes? According to Mark Mattson of the National Institute on Aging-Neuroscience, intermittent fasting generates a slight biological stress that pushes the body to reactivate its cellular defence against molecular damage. According to other experts, however, this would allow the body to detoxify itself, eliminating waste, toxins, and waste products.

Intermittent fasting is a flexible program and allows anyone to follow it. It is an effective way to lose body fat, to preserve lean mass, and to have energy throughout the entire day.

Everyone knows what fasting is, but few people ever experience   it.

Fasting is simply a period of time when you do not eat:

usually, the longest time you do not eat is between dinner and breakfast, so that would be around 10 to 12 hours. It is no coincidence that the Anglo-Saxon countries use the word breakfast, which means "breaking a fast."

In detail, therefore, intermittent fasting (IF) is a diet that alternates phases of fasting (or underfeeding) long (from 16 to 36 hours) and feeding phases. It is simply adding a few hours to the night fast.

There are various types of intermittent fasting: 16 hours of fasting and 8 of feeding at least 2 times a week, 16 hours of fasting and 8 of feeding every day, 24 hours of fasting 1 or 2 times a week (on the day of fasting, only one meal is eaten after 24 hours), 36 hours of fasting, and the Warrior diet (during the day, you can introduce very few calories from vegetables and/or dried fruit, and dinner only consists of just one meal).

When you follow this diet (if in good health conditions and after consultation with your doctor), you may notice health benefits, including the decrease in body weight, decrease in blood glucose levels, increased lipolysis and fat oxidation, and a decrease in food related stress.

Is intermittent fasting good for everyone?

Intermittent fasting should not be followed by those who live the relationship with food in a nervous way, by those who cannot control the amount of food ingested, and by those who continually check the clock to know if they can start eating again.

Before making important choices from the point of view of nutrition, you should always ask advice from an expert, primarily the family doctor—if you are in good health, and a specialist has given their consent, you can try the intermittent fasting road, perhaps starting a little at a time, grouping what you would eat during the whole day in an 8-hour band and fast the remaining 16. The goal must always be 16 hours, perhaps with the tolerance of one hour (15 to 17 hours). As always, before starting any diet or nutritional regiment, we advise you to see your doctor and discuss with him the new approach you want to take.

Why   is   fasting   a   positive   thing?

As reported by Mark Mattson of the National Institute on Aging-Neuroscience, intermittent fasting provides a mild biological stress that drives the body to reactivate its cellular defence against molecular damage. Mice, for example, show higher levels of a protein that protects neurons from death. In this way, Mattson would argue that untimely fasting would remove the risk of stroke and cerebral decline, produce new neurons, and bring benefits to   the   whole   body.

Fasting reduces inflammation, improves the immune system response, enhances the ability of cells to get rid of waste substances, slows the growth of tumours, and reduces the risk of heart disease. The thing that remains important, however, is to continue to drink lots of water. Fasting is not a low-calorie diet—a diet based on fruit or liquid. We do not consume fats, vitamins, or sugar; when you really fast, you do   not   eat   anything   at   all.

In the body, autolysis is then started, which is essentially the process of destruction of worn out tissues. These tissues are replaced by new ones created by the same organism—in short, the body "eats itself" to regenerate itself. In addition to autolysis, fasting accelerates the cleansing of blood vessels, cells, and the environment in which they swim. So now that we have understood the basis of fasting, let's dive deeper into the topic and discover all the secrets of this modern way of eating.

Chapter 2: Why do we eat?

Have you ever wondered why we eat? It is one of those simple questions that is difficult to answer and that has a profound impact on our lives. The first reason why we eat is that it allows us to grow from being an infant until we reach our maturity as an adult. The second function of nutrition is to conserve life. Food gives energy to our body and maintains a caloric level sufficient to conserve the temperature of the body of each species. In this case, human beings have a normal body temperature of 37 degrees Celsius.

What happens if the food is not consumed? The body takes calories from the fat tissue, which is temporarily stored mostly in your belly when you eat. A good health refers to keeping the process of food income and food expenditure in balance. If you eat too much, you go beyond the natural purpose for which fat deposits exist. This will make you obese.

In the richest countries, obesity is an increasingly widespread phenomenon. Various explanations are given as to why there is a widespread obesity in such countries. For some, the impulse to eat beyond measure comes from an ancestral hunger, like if it is a sort of command left in their brain and ready to be activated in the presence of food.

For others, the explanation is found on a psychological level. In fact, we create an abnormal situation with this almost neurotic need for excessive nutrition. Just look at how many mothers overfeed their children today. For example, if you wanted to punish the child for bad behaviour, you would have told him, "As a punishment tonight, you will skip dinner."

A positive food education has been lost.

Today, everything is turned upside down, and it is often the children who threaten their parents not to eat if they do not turn up the television or condescend to their desires. Instead, the golden rule is to eat just a little. Not only because of the cardiovascular risks related to overweight, but also because more food is introduced, and more risks are incurred for cancer. The risk of cancer is proportional to the amount of food that is introduced: more food, huger risk. This is why intermittent fasting is such a powerful concept. In fact, it can be seen as an invitation to frugality and, maybe, to inspire parents to be stricter with their children.

It will certainly be against the current trends, but it is not a secret that many food pathologies are linked to a culture that has lost sight of what really is necessary to survive. Bad diseases such as anorexia and bulimia did not exist almost 30-40 years ago when there was a good education in food and attention to its good use, which was not due to the fact that at that time, it was poorer. As Bismarck said, you can get out of the rules of healthy eating on your birthday, but you do not have to celebrate your birthday every day.

Naturally, eating only once a day should not be understood as a valid model for everyone—not for the sick or for those suffering from particular gastric disorders. Children and pregnant women need more complete nutrition, and people who burn lots of calories for work need to rebalance their energy   expenditure.

Have you ever wondered why fruit looks so aesthetically pleasing? Why there are fruits that tell an unattainable aesthetic perfection and seem to say: you would like to eat me, wouldn't you? And why are the colours of certain fruits also   tempting?
Even this apparently simple question proposes to our attention the mechanism of life on Earth and its conservation and propagation. It is a complex phenomenon, which occurs in a regime of mutual exchange between those that our elementary school books defined, with a suggestive word, the "kingdoms of nature": mineral, vegetable, and animal. The vegetable world absorbs carbon dioxide from the atmosphere and transforms it into plants, which, in turn,   produce   oxygen.

The animal world behaves in the opposite way and is the main character of a reverse project: it absorbs oxygen and burns it, producing carbon dioxide. The Earth lives on this harmonious relationship: on the one hand, plants produce what animals consume, and the product of this process serves the vegetable world to live.

And now, let's go back to the history of mankind. Humans are primates, which means that they are a modified monkey, and the monkey has maintained very basic metabolic characteristics. Primates have been and still are vegetarians and also interact with the plant world because they basically eat fruit.

The flowers, from which the fruit will then be born, are coloured and fragrant because they have to attract pollinating insects that allow fertilization. The fruits, equally coloured and fragrant, attract animals, including humans. However, this harmony and this synergy between different kingdoms and worlds at some point in human history started to suffer from a great problem: the great glaciations. The plants disappeared almost completely. Many vegetarian animals perished miserably.

The human species was saved, and from a vegetarian

species became a carnivore one. The turning point of human nutrition was the ice that covered the planet. Men became carnivorous, but also maintained the metabolism of a vegetarian primate. In short, our organism is programmed for the consumption of fruit and vegetables, and to return largely to this type of food can only benefit us.

We should follow the example of our ancestors' peasants.

What is intermittent fasting?

Although it may seem absurd, fasting is good for the mind and the body. There are many forms of "the fasting diet," but the type that has been rediscovered in recent times is that of intermittent fasting.

The diet varies: from allowing the consumption of calories only for a certain period of the day (usually from six to twelve hours) to drastic caloric reduction for 48 hours— until complete fasting every week.

The studies on intermittent fasting are innumerable, many

19

of which are still "work in progress," but significant benefits are being highlighted on several aspects on a monthly basis.

In addition to losing weight, intermittent fasting would also improve blood pressure and help the body dispose of fat by going   into   ketosis.

Positive indicators also seem to be related to the reduction of cancer risk, especially breast cancer—yet they are still in progress.

Returning to weight, it has been proven that the more the body accuses the fast, the more it uses fat as fuel, thus entering   into   ketosis.

Not only that: there would be a positive feedback as well regarding a significant reinforcement of neural connections with consequent improvement of memory and mood.

Those who practice intermittent fasting report feeling more lucid   and   focused   during   fasting.

Scientists would argue that ketogenic diets would help to fight diseases like Alzheimer's - precisely because of this cognitive improvement at the hands of fasting, which also improves   mood.

Intermittent fasting would seem to be helpful even for diabetes.

A fast that includes, for example, a few days without particular restrictions on food—always following a healthy and controlled diet—followed by a very narrow diet of 5 days, would bring significant improvements to those with high   blood   sugar.

Chapter 3: Basics of Nutrition

Before getting into the details of intermittent fasting, we would like to spend some time talking about the basics of nutrition. It is fundamental to understand the basic concepts, before diving deeper into the topic. When we talk about diet and nutrition, we often do not know the principles that underlie our very existence and, above all, our physical well-being. We limit ourselves to eating something that others have advised us, and we often take pills and tablets advertised, which not only have no use but wrapped up can even be harmful to our health and our finances.

In order not to get lost in the complicated world of nutrition, the first useful thing is to do an overview of food principles and daily human needs.

Let's start by saying that all foods can be classified into five large food groups:

- carbohydrates

- proteins (or protides)

- fats (or lipids)

- vitamins

- minerals

Carbohydrates are the nutrients most present in our diet. They are made up of two main elements—carbon and water —that when joined together give rise to the simplest of sugars, glucose. Aggregating then into larger molecules, they form two different groups of carbohydrates: simple sugars (consisting of a few molecules of glucose) and complex sugars (formed by long chains of glucose). A subsequent classification is that which divides them into monosaccharides (a sugar molecule), disaccharides (two molecules), and polysaccharides (more than two molecules).

There are about 200 different types of carbohydrates, and often times, they take the name from the food in which they are in large quantities. For instance, there are some carbohydrates called fructose, lactose, maltose, but also sucrose and starch. Carbohydrates can be found mainly in vegetables, and their function is purely energetic and makes up the basis of human nutrition—providing about 4 calories per gram/weight. They are found in large quantities in pasta, rice, potatoes, fruit, milk, bread, flour, as well as in legumes.

The cells of our body transform all the carbohydrates introduced into the simplest form, glycogen, which, once oxidized into the cellular mitochondria, provides energy for rapid and above-all clean use, i.e. without waste. These must, therefore, represent the basis of our nutrition and must provide about 60-65% of the energy needs.

However, it is rare to have to carry out a glucosidic supplementation. In fact, they are so widely present in all foods, that perhaps we should think about reducing their consumption.

Fats, on the other hand, are complex acidic structures found in both animal and vegetable foods. Like carbohydrates, fats also have a purely energetic function, with a different caloric value. Lipids bring about 9 calories per gram/weight, and their burning rate is very slow. In fact, before being used, fats must be transformed into simpler elements, which the cell can then oxidize to obtain energy. In their complex form, on the other hand, they are easily stored as fat storage, which is the energy reserve of our body. Fats are often divided into saturated and unsaturated, depending on the type of chemical bond that forms the molecule. To simplify, we can say that saturated fats are "bad" and harmful to our arteries—these include cholesterol, glycerol, hydrogenated fats, fats contained in butter and margarine, palm oil, and most fats of animal origin.

The "good" fats instead are the unsaturated fats or those contained in olive oils and in many seed oils, fish fats (omega 3 and omega 6), and lecithin (abundant in soybeans).

In addition to energy capacity, fats are involved in many organic activities, including hormone synthesis and cell membrane construction. Their function is therefore vital, and our energy needs should be covered by lipids in the measure of 15-20%.

The integration of fats is very rare, as we usually tend to consume more than we should since they are the vehicle of taste and make us better appreciate the foods we ingest.

When it comes to proteins, it is a totally different story. They are composed of complex chains of amino acids joined together by peptide bonds. These amino acids can bind together in number, proportions, and different forms— giving rise to an almost infinite series of specific proteins.

There are 21 amino acids, 8 of which are called "essential," because our body is not able to synthesize them. In fact, human RNA possesses protein synthesis codes for only 13 amino acids and is able to process proteins that contain only these elements. For a complete protein range, it is necessary to take the remaining 8 amino acids, called essential, from the outside through eating.

Animal and vegetable proteins are made of the same amino acids—with a substantial difference. While each animal protein contains all 21 amino acids (in different proportions, depending on the protein itself), in the proteins coming from vegetables, there is always something missing. Some plant foods, therefore, contain certain amino acids but do not contain others. It becomes important, then, in the case of a vegetarian diet, to know how to combine the various products so that all the necessary elements are introduced. As we said, this does not apply to animal proteins, which are called "noble" because they are complete.

From an energetic point of view, protides are similar to carbohydrates, bringing about 4 calories per gram/weight. Unfortunately, however, the energy obtained from proteins is not as clean, because as a result of oxidation at the cellular level, nitrogen is released, which then evolves into free radical, accelerating the cellular ageing process.

The energetic process of proteins is just a fallback of the body in the event of an actual need for calories. Normally, protides are used for "plastic" purposes, i.e. they are used in the construction, repair, and renewal of all body structures —such as muscles, bones, cells, organs, apparatuses, and tissues, in general. It can be said that the human body is composed of 70% water, and the rest of it is proteins. To maintain itself, the human body, therefore, needs a certain daily protein intake, which should be about one gram per kilogram of body weight (a man of 80 kilograms should take 80 grams of protein per day). However, this proportion can range between 0.70 grams per kilogram/weight (the minimum to remain healthy) up to a maximum of 1.5 grams per kilogram/weight. Beyond this threshold, you risk that the proteins are used for energetic purposes would rise to many free radicals and other problems related to kidneys and liver. Ultimately, the daily caloric intake of proteins should be 15-20%.

The supplementation of proteins may be necessary in the case of a vegetarian diet (for the speech of amino acids), while it is almost never recommended in the case of a varied diet that also includes foods of animal origin. Moreover, the assimilation of protides for plastic use is about 4 grams per hour, so we can assume that the body has more means of using them for energy. However, the proteins taken through supplements are less similar than those taken through normal nutrition, as they are metabolized with a certain amount of carbohydrates and vitamins (especially B12).

Another important part of nutrition is the macro group of vitamins. They are organic compounds essential to life and development that normally the human body cannot synthesize and must, therefore, take with food. They are found in large quantities in vegetables, fruit, milk, and its derivatives. Many vitamins are sensitive to high temperatures, so it is advisable to take these foods raw. Moreover, some of them deteriorate over time, becoming bioavailable—this is why it is preferable to eat freshly picked fruits and vegetables.

Each vitamin has a specific function, which can vary from the metabolic one (e.g. B12) to the protective one of the blood vessels (vitamin C). The deficiency of a certain vitamin, usually called avitaminosis, can cause specific diseases, such as scurvy in the case of vitamin C deficiency.

This is why it is important to have a balanced diet in terms of vitamins intake.

Vitamins are distinguished between two categories: water-soluble ones (which means they can be melted in water) and liposoluble ones (melted in fats). Our body is able to store the fat-soluble vitamins (A, D, E, K, and F), while it cannot retain the water-soluble vitamins (C, B1, B2, B5, B6, B12, H, PP) that are easily eliminated in the urine. The latter, in fact, should be taken several times throughout the day. It is also worthy to note that fat-soluble vitamins, which are stored in body fat, have a slower process of elimination. This can cause, in the case of a high intake, a state of toxicity, thus creating very serious dysfunctions. Therefore, if an integration of water-soluble vitamins can be made lightly, we must instead pay maximum attention when it comes to the fat-soluble ones, which should be integrated only in case of established deficiency.

The last food group is one of the minerals and inorganic elements (i.e. without biological carbon) that cover multiple functions. They are often called mineral salts, but this is an improper name since most minerals are devoid of the salt part. Rather, they are single elements present in nature—metals and non-metals—which use water as a vehicle to pass from the earth to the plants and therefore to the animals that feed on them.

They are divided into three groups: macro-elements, micro-elements, and oligo-elements. This division is established on the basis of the daily requirement of the elements, which can vary from 100 milligrams/day for the macro-elements (calcium, phosphorus, potassium, etc.), to less than 200 micrograms/day for the oligo-elements (manganese, chromium, cobalt, etc.).

Although their presence in the body is around 5%/6% of the body weight, they are of vital importance, as they participate in many cellular and metabolic functions. Just think, for instance, about iron, which plays an important part in the cardiovascular system; or calcium, which is a fundamental element of bones and teeth. They must, therefore, be eaten on a regular basis, as the body expels them through the excretory apparatus through urine,

31

faeces,   and   sweat.

A varied diet in which vegetables, fruit, milk, meat, fish, eggs, and dried fruit are added, provides the optimal amount of all the necessary minerals.

Mineral deficiency, just like vitamins, can lead to specific diseases, such as iron deficiency anaemia, or it can even aggravate diseases such as osteoporosis in the case of calcium deficiency. A certain quantity of minerals is therefore vital, but their excess can instead lead to real phenomena of poisoning. Hence, it would be good to stay away from the saline and mineral supplements, unless there's an ascertained shortage. Most importantly, before starting the intake through supplements, it is advisable to seek medical advice.

After reading this chapter, you now have a complete understanding of how nutrition works and how you can use the different elements to create a sustainable meal plan. In intermittent fasting, all the calories will be assumed in a short period of time, but it is still crucial to have a balance ratio of the different nutrients. At first, it all may seem complicated, but once you go through the rest of the book, you will have a much clearer picture of what to do to be successful with intermittent fasting.

Chapter 4: How to Have the Right Mindset

The idea of starting a diet can be daunting, especially if you are not mentally prepared to face such a change. When the mind is calm and prepared, sticking to a healthy food program is much simpler. With the right preparation, you will be able to effectively achieve your goals, and you will make it less difficult not to fall into temptation during the journey.

When it comes to having a good mindset, it is not a secret that it plays an important part on dieting and in the success of the process. Having a positive attitude, will allow to push when things get difficult and to keep the diet sustainable over a long period of time. On the other hand, having a negative thought process can be detrimental to the results. This is why, when starting a diet, like intermittent fasting, it is important to have the right mindset. These are a few tips that will help you along the way. Remember that mindset is 90% of and plays a major role in your success.

Be aware of the recurring negative thoughts related to food.

Often times, our diets fail because of our beliefs related to food and eating. Try to become aware of your food beliefs and make an effort to change your mentality.

We often think that on special occasions, it is right to let go a bit. There's nothing wrong with eating a little more from time to time, but be honest with yourself about what you consider "special occasions." When events like eating away from home, business lunches, office parties, and other small events all become excuses to let yourself binge, the failure of the diet is just around the corner. Try, therefore, to re-evaluate what occasions can be considered as "special" and when it is better to stick to your original diet plan.

Do you use food as a reward?

Many think that after a long busy day, it is normal to deserve to go out for dinner or eat an entire tub of ice cream. Look for alternative ways to reward yourself, which do not include food. For example, take a long hot bath, buy a new dress, or go to the cinema. There are many ways to reward yourself without using food.

Dissociate food from certain activities.

Food is closely linked to numerous rituals. Giving up sugar and fat may not be easy when we emotionally associate them with certain habits. Make a conscious effort to break these dangerous associations.

Try to be aware of the times you eat too much or make bad food choices, both in terms of food and the things you drink. Whenever you go to the cinema, do you buy Coca-Cola and popcorn? Cannot say "no" to a few glasses of wine during the evenings out? Cannot imagine a Saturday morning without coffee and doughnuts? If so, take the extra mile to commit to chopping these associations.

Try changing associations by replacing harmful foods with healthier ones. For example, when you spend the evening out, dedicate it to a board game instead of focusing on drinking. On Saturday mornings, have breakfast with coffee, yoghurt, and fresh fruits. If, at the end of the day, you tend to try to relax through eating, replace the food with a good book or some music.

It is not just about calories.

In the end, you will be more likely to be able to stick to your diet by committing yourself to change your negative behaviours rather than just keeping your calories under control. Try to become aware of when you eat and why you do it. Even if it is only half a biscuit, ask yourself if you are allowing it because you think you have had a bad day. Do you tend to eat because you are hungry or because you feel bored? If you do it out of boredom, try to get rid of this bad habit. Even if you do not exceed the calories, always try to use common sense. Do not eat the wrong foods for the wrong reasons.

Ask for help.

Changing is not easy, and sometimes, we are not able to do

it on our own. Ask for help from friends and family. Let them know you are trying to lose weight, and pray to support yourself. Make sure they know they do not have to invite you to parties where cheap food and alcohol will be served. In addition, ask to be able to vent with them in moments when you will feel particularly frustrated or tempted. Share your goals with all the people living under your own roof.

Establish realistic goals.

Many people tend to sabotage their diet by placing the bar of expectations too high. If you want to be able to stick to your plans, set goals achievable.

Remember that a balanced diet allows you to lose about ½-1 kilo a week, no more. If you intend to lose weight faster than that, prepare to fail.

Initially, you should have cautious goals, so you will be more likely to be able to reach them and have the motivation to continue. Unspecific intentions, such as "This week, eat vegetables every day," and something like, "The next time I eat out of the house, I will order a salad instead of potato chips," are valid starting points that can lead you to the road to success.

Keep a food diary.

If you want your diet to be successful, you cannot exempt yourself from being responsible. Go out and buy a diary that will accompany you along the entire route. Record everything you eat every day and keep a calorie count. A tangible account will force you to notice your bad habits and motivate you to develop new ones.

Plan your meals.

Planning meals and snacks in advance will help you not to give in to temptations. In the days before the start of the diet, make a list of healthy recipes that you intend to prepare. Try to get ahead, for example, by buying or cutting the necessary ingredients. If you want, you can also cook soups and vegetables to keep in the refrigerator—they will be very useful for the first week lunches.

Focus on concrete behaviour.

Limiting yourself to making analyses in abstract terms, it will not be easy to develop greater willpower. Examining your concrete actions will help you start the transformation. Make a list of the wrong habits you want to change. Start with small, gradual changes. Try to commit yourself to abandon an old behaviour for a week, then continue making new changes slowly.

For example, you decide that after work, rather than watching a show, you will walk for 40 minutes. Commit to respecting your purpose for a week. In the following days, you can gradually increase the duration of the exercise, e.g. by walking for an hour. On the occasions when the willpower is not yet sufficient, commit to bringing yourself back to the right path, even if it may mean having to be particularly hard on yourself. Doing so will help you understand that you are the only one who has the power to change your behaviour.

Recognize and admit any failures. Register them on your food diary. Take responsibility for failure.

Describe the reasons that led to failure, highlighting your disappointment. For example, write something like, "At dinner, I ate dessert because I chose to, and I felt guilty after doing it." Although they may sound harsh words, many believe that saying them is useful to express clearly that they have failed. You will feel motivated to make greater efforts to be able to change.

For some, taking a weekly meal "out of the rules" can be a valid help to stay on track. A deprivation that has lasted too long may cause the whole project to go up in smoke. Sticking to a strict diet may seem more feasible when you know that at the end of the tunnel, you can give yourself the coveted food. If you think it might be useful to check you, consider scheduling a premium meal at the end of the week.

Chapter 5: Questioning Your Habits

Eating is a necessary activity—the body is like a car, and without fuel, it cannot work. Unfortunately, however, in our society, overloaded with food and obsessed with dieting, people build a relationship with extremely wrong foods, in which the act of eating becomes an automatic action and too often linked to negative emotions. This chapter will try to explain to you what is the only thing you need to do to improve your relationship with food and make the act of eating an action that will not only bring nourishment but also a pleasure.

Have you ever eaten food without even knowing what you were putting into your mouth?

Do not worry; unfortunately, it happens to many people. Every day, people come to my studio to tell me how they respond unconsciously to their food stimuli, always repeating the same actions and, above all, feeling deprived of   the   strength   to   change.

They tell me how often they do not derive any joy from what they eat and, on the contrary, gain a lot of frustration or guilt from it, and they want to know what they can do to improve their relationship with food. They have often tried everything   and   feel   tired   and   disappointed.

The solution is actually much simpler than what you may believe.

The only thing you need to do to improve your relationship with food is not to do stressful diets (which only lower self-esteem) or spend whole days in the gym, but something much simpler: you have to become more aware of what you are   doing.

Increasing awareness of your automated models can help you make more deliberate food choices and improve your relationship   with   food.

What you have to change is not so much the food you eat,

but more on our relationship with it. Learning to eat with awareness will allow you to understand what your body really needs, and it will allow you to enjoy your meals.

In this way, in the end, you will reach your ideal weight without having to constantly resort to exasperating diets.

How   do   you   do   it?

Simple: you have to learn to be in contact with you! You have to ask yourself some good questions to help you become aware of the hundreds of food decisions you take every   day   without   even   realizing   it.

Here are some good questions you must ask yourself to become more aware and improve your relationship with food.

1.   Why   do   I   eat?

This is the main question that will guide all your future decisions. And in the vast majority of cases, you do not know why you're eating! People hardly stop to wonder what drives them to go to the kitchen and open the pantry drawer. Many times, one believes that they are hungry, but in reality, they only feel like that in response to an emotional stimulus, such as boredom or stress. Learning to recognize this difference is the first step to effectively fight your urges and discover the real needs of your body. Take a break to ask yourself, "Am I really hungry?" Whenever you feel like you need to eat, it will help you differentiate your physical hunger from environmental and emotional stimuli.

2.   When   do   I   eat?

If you have ever followed a diet in your life, you will have realized that the traditional dietary approaches do nothing but provide you with a food plan where they tell you what you should eat, how much you have to eat, and what time you have to eat! This cannot be more wrong. These rules do nothing but disconnect you from your natural nourishment needs and only encourage you to ignore internal signals of hunger   and   satiety.

3.   What   do   I   eat?

Diets are definitely frustrating. They force you to eliminate a lot of things and often the best ones in terms of taste! To be able to do this, you require a certain willpower that must be maintained for a very long time, which is very difficult even for the most persevering people. Learning to consume a little of everything in a moderate way, ranging from healthier foods to those that you eat for pleasure, will lead you to live your relationship with food in a much more balanced way. By freeing yourself from restrictions, you will develop the ability to respond to the wisdom of your body— that innate wisdom that is within each person.

4.   How   do   I   eat?

Quickly? Standing up? Watching TV? Many people eat in a bad way and are so inclined to eat more—this feeling of satiety and satisfaction is, in fact, less when not paying attention to the food you introduce. Learn to avoid multitasking when you eat and dedicate quality time to the activity of eating. In this way, you will be able to feel what your body has to tell you, such as when it is time to stop, so as to avoid the binge you will later regret.

5. How much do you eat?

Normally, classic diets focus on how much you are allowed to eat using methods based on the control of calories or fat. This behaviour, however, in the long run, leads you to spend an enormous amount of time, energy, and willpower. Turning the meal into a mechanical experience will make you disconnect from internal signals, and this will favour problematic behaviours rather than reducing them. Paying attention to the signs of satiety and determining small goals in the situation, such as feeling better after eating than before you start, will make you able to eat the "right" amount of food based on the real needs of your body. For example, young children eat when they are hungry and stop when they are full. They touch, smell, and explore food while eating it. Re-learning these innate behaviours in humans is essential for developing a healthy relationship with food.

Those may seem unimportant questions, but when thinking about them it is easy to understand that they lay the foundation for our relationship with food. It is important to develop a positive view of eating from an early age and if you found that you answered to these questions in a non desirable way, it means that there is some work to do on a psychological level as well.

Chapter 6: Three meals a day is a social construct.

Why do we eat what we eat? The answer suggested by common sense is that we choose to eat what we like. And it is a correct answer: satisfaction is the main factor influencing our food choices. But the question is more complex. Scientific literature has highlighted a link between food and the expression of both social and personal identity —we are what we eat, not only in biological terms but also in symbolic terms. In fact, food practices refer to the different collective belonging and manifest the individual adherence to a lifestyle. Moreover, social psychology, in explaining human behaviour, takes into account the fact that we do not live in isolation but together with other people who inevitably influence us. Therefore, in addition to the tastes and information, we possess (for example, on the presumed healthiness of certain foods), the influence of others also contributes to determining our eating habits, often through identification processes with different social groups. Without claiming to be exhaustive, let's look at some examples of social influence on eating behaviour.

The first to influence us are certainly our parents, especially our mothers, who can condition us in different ways. First of all, through their example: our mothers are the first models we imitate, in general, and also with regard to the relationship with food. Secondly, our mothers even influence the development of our tastes because it circumscribes and delimits our experience with food: our mothers choose the one that enters the repertoire of the foods we come in contact with and selecting the foods to which we are exposed. When we were in their womb, we began to taste and learn about the flavours of our family and our culture. This selective exposure to food continues throughout the period of breastfeeding (even our mothers' milk takes the taste of what they eat) and continues for a long time. In fact, at least until the children reach 11-12 years old, our parents decide which foods come into the pantry and arrive at the table. This type of influence is fundamental because the selection of the food we are experiencing greatly influences our tastes, which are mainly formed through simple exposure and repeated experience. They are built on familiarity—we like what we are used to eating.

A second way by which tastes develop is through associations that are established between a certain food and a positive or negative situation. Parents can also influence these associations: if the family meal is a nice moment and an opportunity for sharing and living peacefully, our relationship with food will be connoted in a positive sense; if the meal is a battlefield, a place of conflict, in which they force us to eat something that does not go well, then our relationship with food will perhaps be compromised and will haunt us even into adulthood.

Growing up, our peers become increasingly important, both in general and as sources of influence, on our eating behaviour. Our peers influence us because we tend to imitate them. For example, at the end of a dinner with new friends, we often ask ourselves: "Should I get the dessert?" It may happen that we have a great desire for it, but if nobody takes it, we will probably give it up. Some research shows that people eat less if they are together with people who eat little and eat more if they are together with people who eat a lot. Why does this happen? In general, there are two fundamental reasons: on the one hand, if we do not know how to behave in a certain situation, which is perhaps new and unusual, we look at what others do to understand what is the appropriate behaviour, and we repeat it; on the other hand, we imitate others because we identify with them because and we want to feel accepted or at least not seem strange or deviant. This is where the idea of having 3 meals a day came from. As we will see in the next chapter, however, it is not the best solution.

Chapter 7: Intermittent Fasting: The Solution

The intermittent fasting diet, invented by Ori Hofmekler, is based on a daily food cycle that includes two phases: underfeeding during the day and overfeeding during the evening-night.

The phase of underfeeding should last all day, applying the rules of the intermittent fasting diet. This naturally stimulates the sympathetic nervous system (SNS) which promotes vigilance, competitiveness, and energy expenditure. During this time, the body moves into a negative energy balance and is therefore forced to burn stored fat to produce energy.

During the underfeeding phase, the consumption of food consisting mostly of raw fruits and vegetables, soups, and small amounts of protein foods should be minimized.

The major food intake phase takes place during the evening-night hours.

This is the moment when the main meal should be consumed when you can eat as much as you want from all the food groups but still following certain dietary patterns, which we will dwell on more later.

Physically active individuals may require more energy and special types of fuel (fats or carbohydrates), depending on the nature and level of their physical activity. The phase of food abundance causes the activation of the parasympathetic nervous system (SNP), which promotes relaxation and recovery.

During this phase, the body moves towards a positive energy balance while creating a general anabolic-constructive state. This is the moment when the body recovers, builds the tissues and fills the energy reserves.

Intermittent fasting takes as an example the soldiers of the

Roman Empire who were subjected to major stresses for wars and large displacements. They were trained to fight and possessed powerful bodies and important muscle masses, so they carried a lot of energy accumulated in the periods   of   rest.

More specifically, the Hofmekler model, which also partly refers to intermittent fasting and caloric restriction studies, provides only one large meal a day after 10-12 hours of fasting or limited to the intake of small protein snacks or fruit   or   vegetable   juices.

Under these conditions, the organism would interpret the fast as a sort of state of emergency and consequently synthesize a whole series of hormones that favour the transformation of fats into energy (growth hormone, adrenaline, noradrenaline) and improve the physical response   to   the   environmental   circumstances.

According to Hofmekler, the fact that breakfast is considered the most important meal of the day has no scientific basis, while the human body would be more alert and efficient if you keep fasting until evening.

Man is, by nature, a nocturnal eater programmed to work and fast during the day and eat and rest during the night, while it would be customary to consume his meals during the day which, going against nature, promotes the development of obesity, diabetes, heart attack, and stroke.

During the day, you will have to eat completely natural foods, such as vegetables, a little fruit, and small amounts of protein.

The goal of the intermittent fasting diet is to create a lifestyle that imitates that of our predecessors from prehistory to ancient Rome (primitives and gladiators).

If we want to summarize everything by giving indications and explanations, we could say that this food model is based on the assumption that nourishing the body by supporting the circadian rhythms of primitive man is functional to the maintenance of physical form and health, as it enhances the use of nutrients and the transformation of body fat into energy while at the same time increasing resistance to stress.

The author has "engraved" the real commandments that "the warrior" subjected to this diet will have to follow. Those are:

- Provide your body with all the essential nutrients (vitamins, minerals, EFA, amino acids, and probiotics). Introduce all the aromas, flavors, textures and colors possible.

- When possible, cyclically rotate the days when carbohydrates, proteins, or fats dominate the caloric percentages taken.

- Avoid foods containing hormones, pesticides, chemical additives, sugar alcohols, artificial sweeteners, and excess fructose.

- Do not eat foods that contain high-glycemic carbohydrates on their own.

- Exercise regularly even during the underfeeding phase.

Avoid wrong food combinations such as:

- Wheat and sugar
- Starch and fats
- Walnuts and parmesan
- Carbohydrates and alcohol

The body is designed to eat this way.

The cyclicity between negative energetic and positive energy balance of genes known as "parsimonious genes" improves human survival chances. This is measured by the ability to improve energy use, performance, and health. Intermittent fasting lets you turn on biological switches that improve human survival day by day.

In the morning, when we just wake up and have an empty

stomach, we have 3 main substances in circulation:

- testosterone – every man has the peak of it in the morning;
- cortisol – a stress hormone, extremely lipolytic hormone; and
- catecholamines — adrenaline and noradrenaline, pure energy.

All these hormones increase energy aggression and mental clarity, and they are stimulated by the empty stomach. In this fasting phase, you will lose weight and water, so it is very important to drink a lot.

If you start eating at this stage of the day, you would raise the insulin and GH levels—hormones that keep you calm, relaxed but little aggressive, lazy, feel weak, and immediately store the energies and lower the 3 hormones above.

The blood then moves away from the muscles to go to the stomach for digestion and therefore less blood to the muscles.

Another positive outcome from fasting is its purification effect on the liver and the kidney.

In the overeating phase, you have to start eating less tasty foods and then move on to tastier foods, so you will start with the intake of salad, vegetables, proteins—then finish with the richest carbohydrate foods.

It will be important to introduce a wide variety of foods—both from the point of view of flavour, consistency, and colour—to get all the nutritive principles (macro and micronutrients).

Intermittent Fasting Meal Plan

The intermittent fasting food plan by Ori Hofmekler is based on a very simple and intuitive structure:

Phase 1 – Low Energy (for about 20 hours)

During the first part of the day, few foods are allowed —mostly of plant origin, such as seeds and simple proteins, i.e. all foods that are not very demanding for our digestive system. This is intended to facilitate detoxification of the body.

The prolonged (but controlled) state of under-feeding triggers physiological processes such as increased insulin sensitivity and increased production of anabolic hormones to counteract the state of "resource shortage" and to make the most of the few present.

Phase 2 – Supercharging (for the remaining 4 hours)

After Phase 1, the body finds itself *emptied* of resources and in a condition of maximum sensitivity to nourishment.

This particular condition makes sure that a large amount of nutrients introduced during supercharging is not lost or "stored" as fat (also due to the low level of insulin).

During this phase, there is no particular constraint on the type of food to be taken or its quantity.

Of course, taking on a diet like this also requires a team of specialists to follow you on the way, since you must not forget that you are a unique biological entity, and as such you will have individual responses that will need specific adjustments to allow optimization of the diet without incurring problems of any kind.

Chapter 8: Different approaches and what to eat

For some time, there has been a total inversion of the currents of thought with regard to the principles of weight loss and the basics of muscular anabolism.

Classic   Approach

Food-induced   Thermogenesis

The fundamentals of "traditional" dietetics suggest losing weight by exploiting also the specific dynamic action of food (ADS), or energy expenditure attributable to digestive, absorption, and metabolic processes.

In practice, with the same calories introduced, with increasing the division of meals, it is possible to burn more energy to process them. This allows you to reduce the amount of time "on an empty stomach" avoiding the "hunger" and keeping the metabolism speedy.

Cortisol and Thyroid Hormones

Some argue that this practice also favours the containment of an unwanted hormone, cortisol (also called "stress hormone") and maintenance of thyroid function (TSH and T3). Obviously, this system works as long as the caloric amount, the nutritional distribution, and the glycemic load-gauges of the meals are appropriate.

Preventing Catabolism

At the same time, in the context of muscle growth, it is (or was) a common opinion that to promote anabolism, it was necessary to "feed" continuously (and "as much as possible," avoiding the increase of fat) muscle fibre cells, in order to cancel any form of catabolism and promote photosynthesis, especially thanks to the insulin stimulus.

What is Intermittent Fasting?

This principle is already heavily inflated and, to be sure,

rather confused. It goes from the "caveman's diet," which involves a huge binge with one or two days of fasting, at the most reasoned "system 16/8" (where 16 is the hours of fasting and 8 is the hours in which 2 or 3 are consumed meals).

The cardinal principle of intermittent fasting is to create a fasting "window" (time lapse) with a duration that affects the overall caloric balance and hormone metabolism.

How   Does   It   Work?

It seems that in conditions of food abstinence, in addition to a total insulin decrease (remember that insulin is a parabolic hormone, but also responsible for fat storage), there is a significant increase in another rather "interesting" hormone: l 'IGF-1 or somatomedin (some also mention an increase   in   testosterone).

The long deprivation of food is then responsible for the secretion of GH (somatotropin), also called "growth hormone" or, more sympathetically, "hormone of wellness."

Unlike insulin, GH, while increasing hypertrophy, does not cause an adipose deposit, but the opposite! That is, it promotes the lipolysis necessary for weight loss. In practice, GH improves "all-around" body composition.

Always in bodybuilding, to increase muscle and decrease fat, it is essential to periodize the diet and training by pursuing distinctly first one and then the other goal. Today, since the intermittent fasting does result in an improvement of the body composition bilaterally (by increasing muscle mass and weight loss), it seems to be the only real solution to all problems.

Example:

Completely avoiding to cite bibliographic sources of dubious reliability (and seriousness), we will describe below the most interesting and undoubtedly best-suited variant that I could read.

First, I stress that despite using the fasting window, the remaining meals cannot be consumed freely. Moreover, to maximize the results of weight loss (and obviously those of increasing muscle mass), it is always necessary to perform the right physical activity.

The protocol differs in 3 daily meals and 1 training session with a fasting window equal to 16 hours.

- 1st meal to be eaten as soon as you wake up: a source of protein and carbohydrates with medium-low glycemic index; few fats
- 2nd meal – breakfast: complete
- Training (bodybuilding or high-intensity training)
- 3rd meal (to be done *immediately* after training) – lunch: complete
- Fasting window from 1:00 pm or 3:00 pm until the following morning.

Obviously, the diet can be adapted to the lifestyle of the subject, but I personally think this is the best solution.

Chapter 9: Practical Ideas on What to Eat

Intermittent fasting is a diet based on the alternation of regular meals and fasting moments, with the aim of speeding up the metabolism and helping to lose weight faster. Here is an example of the benefits and the different patterns of the intermittent fasting diet.

Intermittent fasting is a diet based on the alternation of regular meals and moments of actual fasting. This type of on-off diet allows you to decide, according to different schemes, how to set the above alternation of normal meals and periods of pause from food, which would ensure a positive influence on the calorie balance and hormone metabolism, thus promoting fast weight loss and improving cardiovascular health and the immune system, in general. There are five main examples of intermittent fasting diet to choose from, in which time windows vary between fasting and normal meals, in essence.

Generally, in the examples of intermittent fasting diet, the day can be split in two parts: a fasting phase called fast—which lasts several hours (from 12 to 19-20 hours), in which no food will be introduced with the exception of water, bitter coffee, tea and drinks without sugars—and another part called fed, in which you can eat regularly.

Intermittent Fasting: the 5 Examples of Fasting-based Diets

There are 5 main examples of a diet based on intermittent fasting. Here they are:

Intermittent Fasting

Devised by the athletic trainer Martin Berkhan, this method is based on scheme 16/8, i.e. the division of the day into two parts: 8 hours in which two or three meals can be consumed, and 16 hours of complete fasting.

Eat Stop Eat

This method was devised by the American nutritionist Brad Pilon, which consists of fasting for 24 hours for one or two days a week. In reality, however, in the off days, a basic caloric diet is allowed.

The Warrior Diet

This method, devised by Ori Hofmekler, provides a 4-hour fed phase—distributed between a dinner, where you can eat everything without any restriction of calories or macronutrient intake, and vegetable snacks rich in fiber and dried fruit.

The Fast Diet (or fasting every other day)

Based on the 5: 2 scheme, that is the possibility to eat regularly for 5 days a week and to make a strong calorie restriction in the other two days. In fact, in the off days, there is no actual fasting, but a maximum of 500 calories is allowed for women or 600 for men. The standard two-calorie menu should focus on a hearty breakfast—such as scrambled eggs, ham, and black tea—and a light dinner of fish or grilled chicken and vegetables. Lunch would be missed, while water and herbal teas are allowed throughout the day.

Whole Day Fasting

It is an Eat Stop Eat with one or two days of complete fasting, unlike the diet devised by Pilon. The good news is that in the other 5/6 day,s you can eat ad libitum (as you desire).

Intermittent   fasting: What   to   Eat?

But what to eat in the fed phases of the various intermittent   fasting   diets?

Let us consider as the first example the most frequent type of intermittent fasting, which concentrates the fed phase in 8 hours, followed by a 16-hour fast. Here is a recommended-type menu:

Breakfast
green tea, bitter coffee or herbal tea without sugar, water at will. (This phase is still fasting, considering that these drinks can be consumed safely even in the hours of fasting.)

Lunch (from 12 onwards)
pasta with pesto, mixed vegetables with a spoon of oil, a fruit. (From here begins the fed phase, where you can have meals for the next 8 hours.)

Snack (from 16)
dried fruit 15g, a fruit, 50g of rice or corn cakes

Dinner (at 19)
baked cod, rye bread, mixed vegetables seasoned with a tablespoon of oil, a glass (125 mL) of wine. (Remember to stop the fed phase after 8 hours from the start of your first meal, breakfast excluded.)

This type of menu can also be followed for the 4 hours of fed Warrior Diet, to which is added the possibility of snacks based on vegetables rich in fibre and nuts—as well as for the two-day low-calorie diet Eat Stop Eat but trying to limit the doses, as they are days of reduction and semi-fasting to which they follow 5-6 wherein you can eat freely.

For the Whole Day Fasting Diet, there is no need for any indication, as unlike the previous ones where the fast is partial or relegated to some moments of the day, there are two days of absolute fasting per week, where you are only allowed to drink water, tea, and unsweetened drinks. For the others 5 days, there is no restriction.

Fast diet: what to eat in the 5:2 diet Regarding the Fast diet, or diet every other day, based on the scheme 5:2, i.e. 5 days at full speed and 2 days at caloric restriction, the standard menu for the two days off provides a balance shared between an abundant breakfast and a light dinner that prefers protein foods.

Breakfast
Scrambled eggs, a thin slice of ham, and black tea

Dinner
Fish, chicken, and vegetables (all preferably grilled)

Water, herbal teas, or unsweetened green or black tea at will

Intermittent Fasting: When to Avoid It?

Although it is not such a drastic diet, intermittent fasting is not suitable for everyone. It is, in fact, not recommended for people suffering from diabetes, hypoglycemia, and cortisol imbalance. It is also best to avoid it if you are subject to chronic fatigue or being pregnant or breastfeeding.

What to Eat in Intermittent Fasting: Guidelines

To make the most of your calorie intake on a day of fasting follow these tips:

1) Choose more protein meals that help you feel full longer. Because proteins have enough calories, you cannot take unlimited amounts to reach the maximum limit set by your fasting day, which is 500 calories. However, you can still make proteins the main source of calories.

2) Fill the dish with low-calorie vegetables. They give a sense of satiety, are tasty, and are good for the health. Cook with steam, bake with a teaspoon of oil or sauté in the pan. Then, add some spices or flavourings to prepare a tasty meal. You can also choose to eat raw salad.

3) Keep the carbohydrates to a minimum: they are rich in calories and make you feel hungry quickly. Among the high-carbohydrate foods, you should avoid potatoes, sweet potatoes, pasta, rice, bread,

some fruits (bananas, grapes, melons, prunes, raisins, dates, and other nuts), breakfast cereals, fruit juices, corn-sole-panicle/sweet corn, and anything containing sugar or other syrups.

4) Do not be afraid of healthy fats: although fat is rich in calories, it helps you feel full. Include small amounts of fat in the fasting meal.

Although the recommended caloric intake is 500 calories for women and 600 calories for men, it is not necessary to be really so stiff—but it will be necessary to weigh or measure at least the high-calorie ingredients in your recipes and calculate the calories to avoid overeating the allowed threshold.

A prepared meal can be a solution without too many problems. As with home-cooked meals, look for options that are low in carbohydrates and sugars and rich in protein and vegetables.

What to eat after a fasting period?

Intermittent fasting is the best way to eat for food lovers! In the days of not fasting, you are free to eat whatever you want.

Although, of course, if you want to lose weight, maybe you'll have to limit yourself to eating whatever you want. Additionally, as strange as it may seem, the days where you do not fast probably will help you reduce your appetite instead of increasing it.

You may find that you are not very hungry the day after fasting. You do not need to eat much if you do not want to. It is advisable, instead, to wait to feel the stimulus of hunger before eating on a day when you are not fasting.

Your tastes can change so as to no longer feel the desire for sweet and sugary foods.

You will understand hunger better, and you will feel less the desire to eat snacks. Then, you can develop the ability to wait for meals without worrying about when it will be time to eat.

This kind of changes will not happen immediately: your hunger on non-fasting days can vary greatly. You may find that you are really hungry and eat a lot on the days when you do not fast. Many people experience this in the early days.

Do not worry if this happens; focus only on following your scheduled fasts.

After 6 weeks of fasting, if you still have hunger problems and cannot limit yourself to food and therefore are not losing weight, you may decide to change the method of fasting or make other changes. You should aim to eat normally on days when you are not fasting.

The joy of intermittent fasting is that you can spend most of your free time on food anxiety while controlling your weight and living healthily.

Some people limit their calories on days when they do not fast in an attempt to accelerate weight loss. Although this may work in the short term, it's probably not a good idea in the long run.

If you do not have your normal feeding days, you will probably feel deprived of your favourite foods and develop "diet fatigue."

If intermittent fasting has to become your way of life, it is important that you do it sustainably for a long time.

Scientific studies

Here is a collection of studies that can help you better understand the concepts discussed in the book:

https://www.ncbi.nlm.nih.gov/pmc/articles/PMC3680567/

https://www.ncbi.nlm.nih.gov/pmc/articles/PMC4403246/

https://www.health.harvard.edu/blog/intermittent-fasting-surprising-update-2018062914156

https://newatlas.com/intermittent-fasting-16-8-diet-study-science/55105/

https://newatlas.com/intermittent-fasting-causes-diabetes-debate/54685/

https://www.healthline.com/nutrition/intermittent-fasting-guide

https://www.businessinsider.com/intermittent-fasting-diet-health-benefits-weight-loss-2018-6

https://www.johnshopkinshealthreview.com/issues/spring-summer-2016/articles/are-there-any-proven-benefits-to-fasting

https://sciencebasedmedicine.org/intermittent-fasting/

https://thedoctorweighsin.com/what-science-has-to-say-about-intermittent-fasting/

https://www.popsci.com/intermittent-fasting-science

Conclusion

Thank you for making it through to the end of *Intermittent Fasting: Burn Fat, Lose Weight, and Become Energetic and Happy*! Let's hope it was informative and able to provide you with all the tools you need to achieve your goals whatever they may be. Just because you've finished this book doesn't mean there is nothing left to learn on the topic —expanding your horizons is the only way to find the mastery you seek.

The next step is to stop reading and to start doing whatever it is that you need to do in order to ensure that you are able to create amazing intermittent fasting recipes and dishes. If you find that you still need help getting started, you will likely have better results by creating a schedule that you hope to follow—including strict deadlines for various parts of the tasks as well as the overall completion of your preparations.

Studies show that complex tasks that are broken down into individual pieces, including individual deadlines, have a much greater chance of being completed when compared to something that has a general need of being completed but no real timetable for doing so. Even if it seems silly, go ahead and set your own deadlines for completion—complete with indicators of success and failure. After you have successfully completed all your required preparations, you will be glad you did. For example, you can think about practicing one new intermittent fasting food habit every day, before becoming a general master of the diet. It is your choice, and it is the beauty of dieting and cooking.

Once you have tried the same recipe many times, it is the right moment to invite your friends and ask them to try the intermittent fasting diet—they are going to love it and, best of all, see incredible results with it.

9 781802 532920